OBESITY IN CHILDREN

WHAT YOU MUST KNOW ABOUT CHILDHOOD OBESITY

BY

RAYMOND GRANT

Table of Contents

Chapter one

There is an increase in childhood obesity. It is estimated that about nine million children and adolescents in the United States between the ages of six and 19 are overweight. Obesity is a serious health concern in the world and the diversity of its causes has been a point of serious discussion amongst health professionals. Studies have shown that the said health condition affects children of different socioeconomic status, however, children from lower-income families and members of minority communities are most affected by this issue.

Eating too much isn't the only cause of obesity; hereditary and physiological variables can also contribute. Nevertheless, a lot of kids don't follow the suggested dietary rules for a healthy diet. Roughly 80% of youth are thought to not consume the daily recommended amounts of fruits and vegetables. Children frequently don't consume enough fiber, which could aid in managing weight. Furthermore, a lot of people eat far more calories, fat, and sugar than they need. Sugar-filled drinks, such as juice and soda, contribute significantly to caloric intake. Meanwhile, a lot of kids don't get enough exercise.

A child who is obese is more likely to be overweight as an adult and to be at risk for a variety of diseases and ailments. Additionally, poor dietary habits and exercise regimens are established risk factors for the three main adult causes of death: cardiovascular disease, stroke, and cancer.

What is Obesity in Children?

The state of having more body fat or adiposity than is considered healthy is called obesity. It's a persistent, dangerous illness. It can eventually result in other health issues like diabetes, heart disease, and some types of cancer. Even though obesity is a global health issue, certain nations have higher rates of the disease than others due to a variety of circumstances.

Now that we are aware of what obesity is, let's attempt to address the subject of what childhood obesity is.

A child is considered obese if their weight exceeds what is considered healthy for their height. It is a condition in which a child's health or well-being is adversely affected by excess body fat.

The most often used technique for screening for excess adiposity is body mass index (BMI) calculation. Because body fat varies with age and gender in the US, abnormal BMI cut-offs for children are based on age- and sex-specific percentiles derived from growth charts.

Chapter two

Causes of Obesity in Children

A child may be fat for a variety of causes, such as hereditary or medical ones. However, children who eat unhealthy meals and live sedentary lifestyles are typically overweight. See your pediatrician, who can run testing, if you suspect your child's obesity is related to a medical issue.

Even though there are many different causes of childhood obesity, a few key elements are identified as having a significant role in the epidemic. Among them are:

Poor or lack of physical activities

Environmental factor

Family and Heredity factor

Food Routines

Socioeconomic status

Medication

Health Issue

Poor or Lack of Physical Activities

Today's kids exhibit a decline in their level of general physical activity. Children and adolescents are living increasingly sedentary lives due to a combination of factors including the rising use of computers, longer television viewing sessions, and a decline in physical education in schools.

The epidemic of childhood obesity is mostly being caused by children's increasingly sedentary lifestyles. Children of school age spend most of the day in school, with recess and physical education classes being their only periods of exercise. Physical education was once mandated on a daily basis. Right now Few elementary, middle, and high schools in the United States are required to offer physical education classes every day.

Environmental factor

The environment of today has a significant impact on how children and teenagers develop their habits and worldviews. One major factor is the frequency of television ads that promote unhealthy diets and eating patterns. Children are also exposed to environmental factors that minimize the value of physical activity.

An estimated 40% of food dollars are spent on meals consumed outside the home, such as at athletic events, restaurants, and cafeterias. Furthermore, because portion sizes have grown, people now typically eat more when they go out than when they eat at home. As a result, they eat more calories than they should.

Juice boxes and other carbonated beverages like soda have a significant role in the epidemic of childhood obesity. It is not unusual for a 32-ounce beverage with roughly 400 calories to be sold to youngsters. Children's soda consumption has significantly increased. Research has indicated that every regular soda drinker's daily risk of obesity increases by sixty percent. Sports drinks, boxed drinks, juice, and fruit drinks pose a serious issue as well. These drinks are high in calories, and it is believed that 20% of children who are overweight today are so because they consume a lot of calories from drinks.

Heredity/Family Factor

According to research, childhood obesity may be influenced by genetics. It has been shown that offspring of obese parents are at a higher risk of experiencing similar consequences. An estimated 5 to 25 percent of the risk of obesity is attributed to heredity.

However, a child's susceptibility to obesity or excess weight is not necessarily determined by genes alone. Parental conduct lessons play a significant role. Early on in their child's development, parents should encourage good eating and lifestyle choices, especially if their offspring are at risk for obesity.

Food Routines

The last few decades have seen a substantial shift in food habits.

There has been a significant rise in the average daily calorie intake. In addition, the nutrients required for a balanced diet have been reduced due to the rise in calorie intake.

A significant contributing factor to the development of poor eating habits is food portions. Overeating is on the rise due to the availability of super-size alternatives and all-you-can-eat buffets. In addition to not exercising as much, kids are eating more and burning off less.

Overweight and obesity are conditions that are largely caused by lifestyle and diet choices. Among the most typical ones are:

- consuming a lot of processed or fast food, which is heavy in sugar and fat.

- eating a lot of restaurant meals, which may have higher levels of fat and sugar.

- consuming more food than is necessary.

- excessive use of sugar-filled beverages, such as fruit juice and soft drinks.

- Comfort eating: People who indulge in comfort food may do so for a variety of other reasons, such as low mood or low self-esteem.

Socioeconomic Status

Children and teenagers from households with lower incomes are more likely to suffer from obesity. This is the outcome of various influences influencing actions and behaviors.

Children from lower-income families often cannot afford to participate in extracurricular activities, which leads to a reduction in their physical activity. Additionally, convenience foods—which are higher in calories, fat, and sugar—are frequently chosen by families who struggle to make ends meet and pay their expenses.

An additional factor contributing to the socioeconomic problem of obesity is educational attainment. Parents with low levels of education have not been exposed to knowledge regarding good eating choices and sufficient nutrition. This makes it challenging for them to impart those crucial values to their kids.

Medication

Obesity in children can also be caused by some medications that your doctor may prescribe to treat specific conditions. The following drugs may contribute to childhood obesity:

Glucocorticoids,   including
cortisol

Megace

Sulfonylureas

Tricyclic depression medicines

Inhibitors of monoamine oxidase,
like phenelzine

Diazozolidinediones

Clozapine

Anabolic steroids

Depression-fighting drugs

Medication for diabetes, such as insulin, thiazolidinediones, and sulfonylureas

medicines that prevent seizures, such as valproate and carbamazepine

Health Issues

Some diseases or genetic issues cause some youngsters to grow up overweight or obese. If you suspect that your child's increased weight growth may have a medical explanation, discuss your concerns with their healthcare professional. Among the instances are:

Prader-Willi syndrome: Prader-Willi syndrome is a genetic disease that can result in an insatiable appetite and a metabolism that burns fewer calories than usual. Low sex hormone levels and weak muscle tone are two further signs of the illness. Although there isn't a treatment for the illness, parents can take preventative measures to keep their kids from growing up obese by getting diagnosed early.

Hypothyroidism: Low thyroid gland activity is the cause of the illness known as hypothyroidism. This regulates the rate at which the body burns calories. Children who have hypothyroidism may experience delayed development and sluggish growth. Although it is less frequent than stunted growth and low height in kids, weight gain is common in kids with hypothyroidism. They might also feel exhausted and have pale skin. Treatment for hypothyroidism may involve medications to bring thyroid hormone levels back to normal. The doctor who treats your child can run tests to check for this condition.

Cushing syndrome: Adults between the ages of 20 and 50 are the most common age group affected by this health condition. However, it can occur in kids. The development rate slows down while the rate of weight gain increases in children with Cushing syndrome. Stretch marks, acne, a moon face, easily bruised skin, and exhaustion or depression are symptoms of Cushing syndrome. It is brought on by extended exposure to the body's stress-related hormone, cortisol. The abuse of steroid medications or tumors on the pituitary or adrenal glands may release excess cortisol. Cushing syndrome can be treated with surgery, radiation, chemotherapy, and medications, depending on the underlying cause. Consult your child's healthcare practitioner if you think they could have the condition.

Chapter three

Diagnosis of Obesity in Children

Your healthcare provider may do a physical examination and suggest certain tests in order to identify obesity.

These assessments and trials frequently consist of:

Obtaining the health history of the child

Your medical team may examine your child's past weight, attempts at weight loss, level of physical activity, and exercise routines. You could also discuss controlling your child's appetite and eating habits. Your physician may inquire about previous medical conditions your child has had, medications they use, stress levels, and other health-related concerns. They might also look through the medical history of your family to determine whether your child might be predisposed to any particular ailments.

A comprehensive physical assessment

This includes taking your child's height, monitoring their blood pressure, temperature, and heart rate, listening to their heart and lungs, and looking over their abdomen.

Body Mass Index computation

Your health provider determines your child's body mass index. A BMI of 95th percentile is deemed obese. Risks to one's health are further increased by positions above the 95th percentile. Get your child's BMI measured once a year or more. This can assist in identifying the treatments that may be best for your child as well as their overall health risks.

Determining the waist size

Measured around the waist, the circumference is the measurement. Visceral fat, sometimes referred to as abdominal fat, is fat that accumulates around the waist and may raise the risk of diabetes and heart disease. Waist circumference should be measured at least annually, as much as BMI.

Examining additional health issues

Your medical team will assess any known health issues your child may have. In addition, your healthcare provider will look for additional potential health issues like diabetes, high blood pressure, high cholesterol, an underactive thyroid, liver issues, and high blood pressure.

Your healthcare provider may do a physical examination and suggest certain tests in order to identify obesity.

Chapter four

Why Obesity in Children is a problem: Health risk associated with Obesity

As you are aware, being overweight can lead to a variety of health issues, particularly in young patients who may experience asthma attacks, sleep apnea, problems with their bones and joints, type 2 diabetes, heart disease risk factors, hypertension, early puberty, and orthopedic issues.

Overweight or obese children are more prone to experience bullying, which can result in eating disorders, behavior issues, learning difficulties, and social isolation in addition to a diminished sense of self-worth. Lastly, obese children are more likely to stay that way as adults, which puts their health at increased risk for conditions like cancer, diabetes, and heart disease.

Compared to their classmates who maintain a healthy weight, children who are obese are more likely to experience health issues. Among the most dangerous conditions are diabetes, heart conditions, asthma, sleep disorders, and joint pain.

Diabetes

A person with type 2 diabetes has improper glucose metabolism in their body. Diabetes can affect the proper functioning of the kidneys, nerves, and even the eyes. Type 2 diabetes is more likely to develop in children who are overweight. On the other hand, dietary and lifestyle modifications might be able to reverse the illness.

Heart Conditions

Children who are obese have a higher chance of developing heart disease in the future due to excessive blood pressure and cholesterol. Foods heavy in fat and salt have the potential to raise blood pressure and cholesterol.

Heart disease can lead to two potential complications: heart attack and stroke.

Asthma

Chronic lung inflammation is known as asthma. Though the precise mechanism underlying the association between obesity and asthma is unknown, obesity is the most common comorbidity with asthma. Studies have indicated that approximately 38% of adult Americans who suffer from asthma also have obesity. The same study discovered that while not all obese individuals have more severe asthma, some may be at risk for it.

Disorders of Sleep

Obese children and teenagers may also experience sleep disturbances like sleep apnea and loud snoring. An excess of weight around the neck may obstruct their breathing.

Joint Aches

Carrying too much weight might also cause your child to have a restricted range of motion, joint stiffness, and pain. Most times, joint pains related to obesity can be averted when the person's weight is decreased.

They may also experience emotional and social issues such as:

Uncertainty
Low regard for oneself
Depression
Mistreatment

Chapter five

Treatment of Obesity in Children

Treatment of obesity in children is based on the child's age and any additional medical issues if any. Treatment typically entails dietary and exercise modifications for your child. Treatment options in some cases may involve drugs or bariatric surgery.

Children whose Body Mass Index falls between the 85th percentile and 94th percentile

Children are deemed overweight if their BMI is in the 85th to 94th percentile range. In order to halt the progression of weight gain, the American Academy of Pediatrics advises placing children older than two who weigh in the overweight range on a weight-maintenance program. With this tactic, the youngster can gain inches but not pounds, which eventually lowers the BMI into a healthier range.

Children whose Body Mass Index is at the 95th percentile or above

Obese children have a BMI that is at or above the 95th percentile. Children who are obese and between the ages of 6 and 11 may be encouraged to change their eating habits to lose weight gradually—no more than one pound per month. It may be recommended for older kids and teenagers who are obese or severely obese to change their eating habits in order to lose up to two pounds every week.

The same techniques apply whether your child is trying to maintain or reduce weight: In addition to increasing physical activity, your child has to follow a healthy diet that is balanced in terms of food types and quantities. Your dedication to assisting your child in making these changes will determine how successful they are.

Healthy diets/eating

It is the parent's responsibility to shop for goods, prepare meals, and choose dining locations. Your child's health can benefit greatly from even modest adjustments

Increase your fruit and vegetable intake: Reduce your consumption of convenience foods, which are frequently heavy in sugar, fat, and calories, such as cookies, crackers, and prepared meals, when you go grocery shopping.

Reduce your intake of sugary drinks Fruit: Juice-containing beverages fall under this category. These drinks provide a lot of calories but not much nutritional benefit. Additionally, they may cause your child to feel too full to consume healthful meals.

Steer clear of quick food:

The majority of the menu items are heavy in calories and fat.

Share meals as a family:

Make it an occasion to exchange news and tales. Avoid eating in front of a computer, TV, or video game screen as this can cause you to consume quickly and become less conscious of how much you are eating.

Serve sensible serving sizes: Compared to adults, children don't require so much food. If your child is still hungry after starting with a little piece, they can ask for more. Even if your child has to leave food on the plate, let them eat only until they are satisfied. Additionally, keep in mind that restaurant portions are frequently far too large while dining out.

Physical activities

Physical activities have a vital role in reaching and sustaining a healthy weight, particularly for children. Besides helping kids sleep better at night and remain awake throughout the day, it burns calories and improves bones and muscles.

Adolescents who develop healthy habits as children are more likely to maintain a healthy weight. Again, kids who are active grow up to be fit adults.

How to get your kids more active

Cut down on screen time:

For kids older than two, recreational screen time—whether it be on a TV, computer, tablet, or smartphone—should be restricted to no more than two hours per day. There should be no screen time for kids under the age of two.

Place focus on activities rather than exercise alone:

Kids should be active for at least

an hour a day, ranging from mild to strenuous. The goal of your child's activity should simply be to get him or her moving; an organized exercise regimen is not necessary. Playing games like jump rope, tag, or hide-and-seek can be excellent for increasing physical fitness and burning calories.

Discover what your child enjoys doing:

If your child has artistic tendencies, for example, take them on a nature hike where they can gather pebbles and leaves to create a collage. If your kid enjoys climbing, take them to the closest climbing wall or jungle gym in the area. If your child enjoys reading, take them for a book from the local library by bike or walking.

Medication

Medication may be recommended for certain kids as part of a weight-loss regimen. Only certain circumstances warrant the prescription of medication, such as in the case of children with diabetes, obesity, or other illnesses linked to obesity.

Operation or Surgery

Adolescents with extreme obesity who have not been able to lose weight with lifestyle modifications may consider weight-loss surgery as an alternative. However, there are possible hazards and long-term complications with any procedure. Talk about the benefits and drawbacks with the pediatrician.

If the possible dangers of surgery are outweighed by the health danger that your child's weight poses, your doctor may advise this operation. A kid who is being considered for weight-loss surgery should have a consultation with a multidisciplinary team of pediatric doctors, which should include a dietician, psychologist, and an expert in obesity medicine. Surgery for weight loss is not a miracle treatment. It does not ensure that a teenager will shed more pounds or be able to maintain the weight off in the long run. Furthermore, surgery cannot take the place of a balanced diet and frequent exercise.

Chapter six

How to Manage Obesity in Children

A family doctor or pediatrician should perform a comprehensive medical evaluation on any obese youngsters to rule out any physical causes. The doctor can advise starting with changing the child's dietary choices and upping their physical activity level if there isn't a physical illness. Making good food and regular exercise a family activity might increase the likelihood that the child or adolescent will successfully control their weight, as obesity frequently affects multiple family members.

Among the strategies for managing childhood and teenage obesity are:

- Seek out expert assistance

- Consult a dietitian to help you modify your eating habits.

- Prioritize well-being as a family.

- Reducing the likelihood of shame can be achieved by speaking positively and offering lots of support.

- Ensure that your youngster is getting adequate sleep.

- Plan your meals and choose several options.

- Monitor what your child eats at school.

- If you're short on cash, ask for assistance choosing a range of foods.

- Boost physical activity, particularly when it comes to

sports or active playing for kids.

Often, obesity develops into a chronic problem. Because obesity requires children, adolescents, and families to adopt new habits, which is difficult for anyone to achieve, obesity becomes a chronic or lifelong problem. It is necessary to incorporate new food and exercise habits into daily life. The expense of food and living in an unsafe environment are just two examples of the many external factors that may make overcoming obesity even more difficult. By concentrating on their child's good traits and strengths instead of merely their weight, parents of obese children can help their children feel better about themselves.

A child and adolescent psychiatrist can collaborate with the child's family physician to create a thorough treatment plan when a kid or adolescent with obesity also experiences emotional difficulties. Reasonable weight loss objectives, diet and exercise control, behavior modification, and family engagement would all be part of this plan.

Teach Children Healthy Eating Habits

Do not advocate diets or limited eating patterns for weight loss if a doctor or nutritionist has not recommended them for medical reasons. Young adults need to eat a balanced, healthful diet. Serving nourishing meals and snacks that are full of a range of colorful fruits, vegetables, whole grains, lean meats, and healthy fats are some helpful ideas to promote and foster healthy eating.

Avoid sugary drinks such as soda and sports drinks.

Kids should help prepare meals.

Include snack time in your everyday schedule.

Eat not in front of a screen.

Take note of the children's eating habits when they are not at home.

By doing these frequently your child gets the awareness of what to eat and what not to eat, how to eat, and when to eat.

Summarized tips for parents

A nutrition plan and objectives for improved physical activity and healthy weight loss are recommended by the healthcare professional once a child receives an obesity diagnosis.

The majority of experts advise following the following broad guidelines:

The decision of what to buy, how to prepare, and when to consume it must be made by parents, not by the kids.

1. A balanced diet should include lots of fresh produce, lean meat, whole grains, avocados, and healthy fats like olive oil.

2. The diet should be cleansed of processed meals, fried foods, high-calorie/high-sugar drinks, sugary baked

products, trans fats, and saturated fats.

3. Nuts, fresh fruits, and whole foods high in fiber like popcorn are good choices for healthy snacking.

4. Parents should steer clear of eating out, especially at fast-food establishments, and prepare as much as possible at home.

5. Family dinners should be shared with plenty of time for

conversation between parents and kids.

6. Eating in front of the TV or while using any kind of electronic device—including smartphones—should be prohibited by parents. Research has indicated that eating while playing video games or watching television can lead to overeating and eating too quickly.

7. In order to avoid the common mistake of making their child finish everything on the plate,

parents should supervise their children's portion sizes.

8. Parents should be aware that restaurant meals are typically far too large while dining out. Consider dividing the dish and packing up half for a future dinner at home.

9. The amount of time a child spends watching television and playing video games is something parents should restrict.

10. Parents should support their children's play-based physical activity, including riding a bike, for at least an hour every day.

Chapter seven

Childhood Obesity and Stigma: An Issue that Must be Addressed

Obese people experience a persistent and widespread kind of social stigma that is upheld and encouraged by society. For a long time, the condition of obesity has been understood to result from an individual's bad eating and movement habits. People who are obese are frequently portrayed in dehumanizing and demeaning ways in entertainment and cultural standards. They are frequently shown as eating excessive amounts of unhealthy food or in unattractive ways. In actuality, it is a multifactorial, intricate illness that is influenced by genetic, epigenetic, physiological, environmental, and socioeconomic factors. Obese children shouldn't face discrimination. It is not their fault or choice that they have the body they do.

No child should ever have to endure the unfavorable opinions of others due to anything, including their weight. Nonetheless, there are unfavorable perceptions about obese persons of all ages. even with kids.

The prevalence of childhood obesity is increasing. More kids will experience the detrimental impacts of stigma and weight bias. It might be difficult enough for a child to deal with the negative health impacts of obesity. Unfair treatment can only make their life more difficult.

Obese children and teenagers experience a variety of weight stigmatization tactics, such as verbal and physical abuse, social isolation, physical bullying, and differing expectations from adults.

We refer to name-calling, disparaging comments, making fun of someone, etc. as *verbal teasing*.

We define *social exclusion* as being ignored, excluded from peer activities, subjected to rumors, and subjected to cyberbullying on social media.

Physical bullying includes pushing, shoving, kicking, and other similar actions.

What Effect Does Children's Weight Stigma Have?

Children who are overweight experience severe stigma related to their weight. They become more susceptible to worry, despair, low self-esteem, and negative body image. According to studies, children who are obese and experience negative attitudes from their peers are more likely than other children to have suicidal thoughts and behaviors.

Experiences with weight stigma might lead to health issues. These consist of binge eating, bad eating habits, and attempting unhealthful weight-loss techniques. A child's heart health may also be impacted by weight bias. Teens who experienced unjust treatment because of their appearance, according to one study, had higher blood pressure even after controlling for factors including gender, exercise level, posture, mood, and current body weight.

A child's overall quality of life is significantly diminished by the additional impacts of weight prejudice, reductions in social and emotional well-being, educational performance, and physical and psychological health. Weight bias has an impact on a child's life in every aspect.

How can the stigma around weight be addressed?

It takes all of us working together to combat weight stigma. There are numerous ways to become engaged, from little everyday acts to advocacy initiatives like contacting legislators. Here are a few instances of how you can contribute to these initiatives.

- Be considerate while addressing those who are impacted by obesity. When discussing someone else's weight, use tact and consideration in your language. One technique to teach others how to use polite language is to set an example for them.

- If you see someone's weight being made fun of, speak up. Jokes about obesity are not funny; rather, they hurt people and perpetuate the stigma in society. Inform your loved ones that their acts are unjust and upsetting if you are the victim of weight bias.

- Inform the people in your life about the negative effects of weight stigma. Reducing damaging weight-based stereotypes can be achieved by educating people about obesity as an illness with multifaceted causes.

- If your children are in school, find out if their school has an anti-bullying policy. Does it favor children with obesity? If not, you can bring up this matter with administrators at the school.

- Is there a policy against harassment in place at work? Is

there a way to make this policy better so that obese employees won't be subjected to discrimination or mistreatment due to their size?

- Tell your doctor or other healthcare practitioner about any instances of weight bias you experienced while receiving treatment. This may encompass how healthcare providers have discussed your weight with you.